The *Natural*
Way To

CONTROL HYPERACTIVITY

With Amino Acid and Nutrient Therapy

by **Billie Jay Sahley, Ph.D.**
Author of *The Anxiety Epidemic*
and Breaking Your Addiction Habit

Pain & Stress Therapy Center Publications
San Antonio, Texas
1994

Note to Readers

This material is not intended to replace the services of a physician, nor is it meant to encourage diagnosis and treatment of illness, disease, or other medical problems by the layman. This book should not be regarded as a substitute for professional medical treatment and while every care is taken to ensure the accuracy of the content, the author and the publishers cannot accept legal responsibility for any problem arising out of experimentation with the methods described. Any application of the recommendations set forth in the following pages is at the reader's discretion and sole risk. If you are under a physician's care for any condition, he or she can advise you as to whether the program described in this book is suitable for you or your child.

This publication has been compiled through research resources at the Pain & Stress Therapy Center, San Antonio, TX 78229.

The names of the patients described in this book have been changed to protect their privacy.

First Edition, Watercress Press, 1988
Second Edition, Pain & Stress Center Publications, 1994

Additional copies may be ordered from:
Pain & Stress Therapy Center
5282 Medical Drive, Suite 160, San Antonio, Texas 78229-6043

Library of Congress Catalog Card Number 93-87629
ISBN 0-9625914-3-2

Contents

Acknowledgments

My sincere appreciation and thanks to:

The staff of The Pain & Stress Therapy Center of San Antonio, Texas (past and present) for their support and dedication to helping children.

Antonio L. Ruiz, M.D, Medical Director of The Pain & Stress Therapy Center for his support and encouragement, and contributions to the understanding of God's natural healers within the body.

Dr. Jeffrey Bland for his support, interest and encouragement in education for optimal health.

Dr. Katherine M. Birkner for her scientific collaboration which helped make this book possible.

Doris Rapp, M.D., one of God's gifted healers, and an inspiration to those who reach out to the hyperactive children of the world.

Dedicated . . .

To the many parents of hyperactive children who believed in me and encouraged me to continue my research to show the importance of amino acids and nutrients on the brain and behavior.

To my associate, Dr. Katherine M. Birkner, for all of the unselfish hours of research spent with me at the University of Texas Health Science Center Library in search of information presented in this book.

And to the new generation of physicians, therapists and educators who seek a natural alternative through nutritional medicine.

And to the Lord for always lighting my path.

Introduction

Orthomolecular therapy means supplying the cells with the right mixture of nutrients. Many diseases are known to be the result of the wrong balance of essential nutrients in the body. Adjusting the diet, eliminating junk foods and ingesting the proper doses of essential vitamins, minerals and amino acids, can correct the chemical imbalance of disease.

The orthomolecular approach helps patients become more aware of our dangerously polluted environment and nutrient-stripped refined foods. The orthomolecular approach is both corrective and preventative. Meganutrient therapy has become a part of orthomolecular medicine. While it is becoming widely recognized that orthomolecular therapy cures patients by correcting brain chemical imbalances, it is little known that in certain combinations meganutrients can be as immediately effective as potent pain-killers or tranquilizers. Meganutrients treat the whole person's biochemical imbalances; they can be of immediate and long term benefit. The type of treatment offered by orthomolecular doctors and therapists varies, but the mainstream of work focuses upon meganutrient therapy and diagnostic tests, and treatment with adequate nutrients is a distinguishing characteristic of orthomolecular medicine.

Orthomolecular therapy takes into consideration that every individual is biochemically unique. Every patient has a very different nutrient and amino acid requirement, and with application of this therapy, each individual's need is met, and the mind and body are in a state of homeostasis--a condition where everything in the body is in balance and capable of resisting environmental changes, while regulating internal metabolic function.

Every tissue of the body is affected by nutrition. Under conditions of poor nutrition the kidneys stop filtering, the stomach stops digesting, the adrenals stop secreting, and the other organs follow suit.

Good nutrition is the preservation of health and prevention of disease--especially with respect to the question of the optimum intake of essential vitamins, minerals and amino acids.

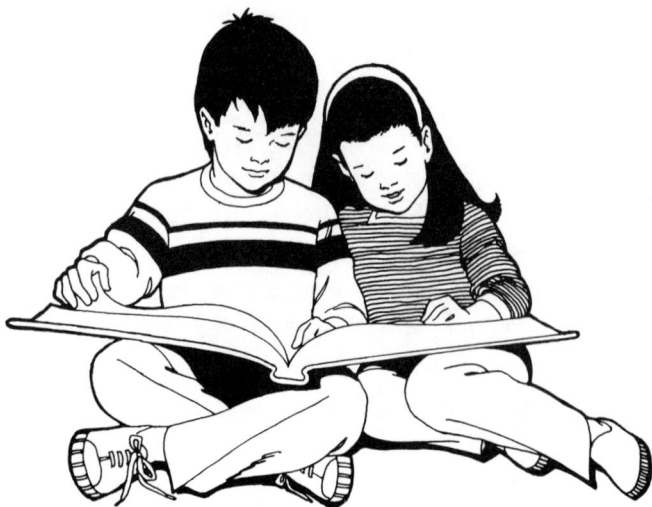

Controlling Hyperactivity With Amino Acid and Nutrient Therapy, Not Drugs

There are approximately 6 million children in this country who suffer some type of learning disability, hyperactivity, A.D.D. (Attention Deficit Disorder) or hyperkinesis. More than one million children are currently taking Ritalin for hyperactivity and A.D.D. Hyperactivity is often caused by physiological disorders such as nutritional and chemical imbalances, blood sugar disturbances, allergic responses to food and chemicals, or a poor diet. Hyperactivity may also result from organic brain dysfunctions, but we will focus on the physiological disorders that cause hyperactivity.

Ritalin is a potent stimulant available only by a physician's prescription. The prescription rates for Ritalin have doubled between 1985 and 1989. The United States Drug Enforcement Administration lists five grades of controlled substances based on abuse potential. Heroin and LSD are "Schedule I." Schedule II drugs include morphine, opium and Ritalin, and yet this potent drug is being used as a quick fix to quiet or calm children down.

Children who show signs of hyperkinesis, hyperactivity or Attention Deficit Disorder that *could* have an imbalance in their brain's biochemistry. A biochemical imbalance that goes untreated can cause a child to display hyperactive behavior, and may result in physical illnesses as well. Through continued research by members of the Academy of

Orthomolecular Medicine and prominent researchers such as the late Carl Pfeiffer, M.D., Jeffrey Bland, Ph.D., and Doris Rapp, M.D., we now know that, hyperactive behavior and certain learning disabilities can be treated by orthomolecular therapy.

A child's state of health is their state of nutrition. When minerals, vitamins, amino acids, enzymes, or even hormones are deficient in a child's system, the result can be a disturbed biochemical homeostasis causing impaired functions in his brain.

The Safe Alternative

At the Pain and Stress Therapy Center in San Antonio we have successfully treated children with meganutrient therapy that corrects the brain's biochemical imbalance. This is done without toxic drugs that produce adverse side effects. The child's biochemical imbalance is corrected by meganutrient therapy which can effect both short term and long term benefits, and is both corrective and preventive. Children are given a complete evaluation, which includes food sensitivity screening and blood work, and a behavioral analysis. The child's progress is charted on a regular basis. The children are provided with dietary reforms, amino acids, vitamins and special nutrients to enhance the optimum molecular environment for their mind and body.

Hyperactivity is a major problem facing parents today. Most people think of hyperactivity as some type of behavioral problem--a child who is impatient, impulsive and constantly moving, but not all children who are hyperactive are aggressive. Some are very passive, withdrawn, and find it hard to communicate their feelings.

Let's examine the list of passive and aggressive behavior and see exactly where your child might fit in. Some children have more than one of these symptoms--they have both

Behavior Symptoms Of Hyperactivity Or Attention Deficit Disorder

Aggressive Behavior	Passive Behavior
Angry outbursts	Depressed moods
Quarrelsomeness	Anxious
Aggressiveness	Fearful
Restlessness	Stays close to mot her
Stealing	Mood swings
Resentment of punishments	Sleep problems
Unaware of danger	Withdrawn
Inability to concentrate	Accident prone
Self-mutilation	Emotional instability
Compulsive aggression	Distractibility
Clumsiness	Slow reader
Not good in sports	Poor math calculations
Temper tantrums	Temper tantrums
Unable to complete projects	Daydreams
Junk-food eater	Eating problems
Eats lots of sugar and drinks a lot of caffeine	Poor muscle coordination
Poor muscle coordination	Lying
Lying	Skin problems such as rash or hives
Poor sleep habits	Reasoning difficulty
Poor handwriting, drawing, and reading skills	Poor reading skills
Show-off	Hyperventilates
Bully	Showoff
Inability to make and keep friends	Poorly developed musculo-skeletal system
	Insecurity

passive and aggressive behavior--but some exhibit only passive *or* aggressive.

Keeping a Daily Record

If your child demonstrates any of this behavior, then you must examine *all* of his habits, keeping a daily log which will prove to be invaluable in therapy. It's like a puzzle, and you are putting the pieces together with one goal: a happy, healthy child who is free of drugs.

Hyperactivity is not a condition that can be measured in precise scientific terms. Nor is it a situation that has a quick fix, especially with a powerful and addictive drug such as Ritalin. Hyperactivity is a behavioral complex in which the child demonstrates maladaptive or disorganized behavior characteristics which puts him out of sync with the world around him. Hyperactive children are extremely vulnerable to other people and to their own inadequacies. Given this information, you must take into consideration his environment as well as possible food sensitivities and allergic reactions to foods, chemicals and poor diet.

Allergic Reactions

Doris J. Rapp, M.D., Pediatric Allergist, who treats many hyperactive children, describes in her new book, *Is This Your Child?*, medical symptoms which are due to allergic reactions that you might observe in your child. Dr. Rapp refers to this as the "allergic-tension-fatigue syndrome." The medical symptoms include:

Nose: year round stuffiness, watery nose, sneezing, nose rubbing.

Aches: head, back, neck, muscles, joints, growing pains or aches unrelated to exercise.

<u>Belly</u> <u>problems</u>: belly aches, nausea, upset stomach, bloating, bad breath, gas stomach, belching, vomiting, diarrhea, constipation.

<u>Bladder</u> <u>problems</u>: wetting pants in the daytime or in bed, need to rush to urinate, burning or pain with urination.

<u>Face</u>: pale, dark eye circles, puffiness below eyes.

<u>Glands</u>: swelling of lymph nodes of neck.

<u>Ear</u> <u>problems</u>: repeated formation of fluid behind eardrums, ringing ears, dizziness, excessive perspiration, and low grade fever.

Dr. Rapp also states some children are fatigued, tired, weak, mentally confused, irritable, drowsy, depressed, have body aches, fever, chills, and night sweats. These children often sleep poorly, awaken at night, have nightmares, and cry out in their sleep. And often these children have learning problems.

Using this information as a guideline, watch your child's behavior for one week, to see what he or she does and how he or she acts in specific situations. At the same time add to your log what he eats--especially how much sugar and caffeine he consumes.

Sugar Addiction

Dr. Janice Phelps, in her book, *The Hidden Addiction and How to Get Free,* says sugar addiction causes many insidious symptoms that are not recognized right away. Gradually, addicted people recognize that they do not feel as good as they should. Children can have extreme reactions to sugar such as aggressive behavior, constant movement and incessant talking. When withdrawn from sugar and supported with complex carbohydrates and the proper amino acids, vitamins, minerals and protein, they show marked improvement.

Dr. Phelps goes on to say sugar addiction is the world's most widespread addiction and the hardest one to break. "Sugar addiction" refers to both refined sugar or simple carbohydrates. Complex carbohydrates break down more slowly so they enter the system slower and do not invoke hyperactive symptoms like the simple ones do.

Because sugar addiction is so widespread and is shared by so many addictive children as well as adults, Dr. Phelps believes it is the "basic addiction" that precedes all others. Sugar dysmetabolism is a major factor in the profile for addiction. Sugar addiction can last a lifetime, or the sugar addict may progress to other addictive substances such as alcohol, street drugs or prescription drugs.

The following are a few examples of the sugar content of foods:

Food	Sugar Content
12 ounces cola drink	12 teaspoons
12 ounces chocolate malt shake	18 teaspoons
1 cake donut	4 teaspoons
1 cup vanilla ice cream	7 teaspoons
1 piece apple pie	15 teaspoons
1 cup sugar coated cereal	8 teaspoons
1 white flour waffle, plain	5 teaspoons
1 chocolate eclair	10 teaspoons

Most addictive people suffer at least some other symptoms as a direct result of their disturbed carbohydrate metabolism. Children who are addicted to sugar go through mood swings--false highs then lows. As they get older they are more likely to try drugs. The sugar makes them predisposed to addiction.

The amino acid, glycine, has been used successfully to help break a sugar addiction. Glycine also has a calming effect as it is an inhibitory neurotransmitter in the brain. For example, one of our patients was a nine year old boy who was hyperactive but responded to amino acids. But he would still crave something sweet from time to time after school. A 250 mg capsule of pure glycine was given to him by sprinkling it on a half piece of fruit or on an oat bran muffin. His mother reported Donnie was completely satisfied with this.

Recently, at the Pain and Stress Therapy Center, I saw a girl named Julie--an 11 year old whose parents were concerned about her behavior. Her teacher had told them she was hyperactive. I asked her parents to take all sugar products out of her diet and as they eliminated them, write down the product name and how much sweetener was included. (That information is usually on the side of the box.) The next time I saw Julie, her mother and I figured out she was consuming in the range of 20 to 25 teaspoons of sugar per day. The best part was yet to come. After we ran a complete blood study and dietary evaluation on Julie, Dr. Ruiz noted high triglycerides and cholesterol--especially for an eleven year old child. Julie was placed on an orthomolecular supplement program and scheduled for behavioral modification therapy.

After three weeks the difference was almost unbelievable. Julie was happy and smiling, and sat quietly and read a book while I spoke with her mother. Then the bomb fell, her mother informed me that Julie's teacher insisted she be put on Ritalin when she went back to school. Julie's mother heard other parents talk about their children's change when they were placed on Ritalin and all of the adverse side effects, besides being extremely addicting. She was so right!

As we have mentioned earlier, not only is Ritalin addicting, but it is also a Schedule II drug, in the same class with morphine and opium. Yet doctors are prescribing Ritalin for our children without a second thought.

Julie did not need Ritalin, she needed specific nutrients in her brain to establish her molecular balance.

The Responsibility of Teachers

Too many teachers find it easy to tell a parent, "Your child is disrupting my class--maybe they should be put on Ritalin." Teachers, *especially*, need to be educated about natural alternatives and nutrient deficiencies. They should be asked whether they would put their child on Ritalin?

Latest records from the manufacture of Ritalin indicate up to 1 million children are now taking it on a regular basis. A report in the *Journal of the American Medical Association*, October 21, 1988, discusses a survey done of school nurses in all of the county and private schools in the Baltimore area to determine the prevalence of medication treatment for hyperactivity / inattentiveness. Among students, the results reveal a consistent doubling of the rate of medication treatment for hyperactivity and inattentive students every four to seven years. The report shows 5.96% of all public elementary school students were receiving such treatment.

"In the late 1980's, the stimulant medication treatment of U.S. children has returned to become a noteworthy public issue (*New York Times*, May 5, 1987, p. 3 and *The Reporter Weekly*, September 2, 1987, p. 10). If present trends continue, over 1 million U.S. children will be receiving stimulant medication by the early 1990's, with possibly one fourth of these children receiving the medication for inattentiveness associated with a learning impairment." The report continues to make an additional statement, "In view of this, additional public health oriented assessment research should be funded. As a result more specific guidelines for physicians may need to be recommended!"

An editorial in the same journal states Attention Deficit/ Hyperactivity Disorder represents one of the most common and serious neurobehavioral disorders of childhood affecting children from early childhood into adult life. Over the 16 year period, stimulants, primarily methyophenidate hydrochloride (Ritalin), came to be used exclusively in the treatment of hyperactivity. The editorial goes on to point out that children are given Ritalin for inattentiveness rather than hyperactivity. This has caused a constant rise in the number of prescriptions. But inattentiveness is a completely different problem and does NOT require Ritalin. This editorial was written by Sally Shaywitz, M.D. and Bennett Shaywitz, M.D. of Yale University School of Medicine.

Ritalin's Side Effects

Side effects of Ritalin have been reported to range from headaches, insomnia, and loss of appetite to anorexic behavior, stunted growth, memory loss, hostility, and even suicidal behavior. In some cases, the child becomes violent with everyone. No doubt at this point, drug sales for hyperactive children is a very big business. Even though Ritalin may be used effectively as a temporary tool in a very difficult situation, it should *never ever* be considered a final method. Its tragic that very young hyperactive or inattentive children are sometimes placed under the care of a chemical baby-sitter or a chemical straight jacket, and not just for months but for years.

Dr. Steven E. Breunig of the University of Pittsburgh Medical School, and a leading researcher on drug use with mentally retarded children, has shown that more than 20 percent of the children taking major tranquilizers or stimulant type drugs will develop permanent tardive dyskinesia. This is a serious disorder characterized by epileptic type movements of the mouth, arms, neck and trunk. Dr. Breunig has also shown that the drugs can impede the child's ability to learn, cause blood disorders, eye problems, suppress appetite, create insomnia and generally dampen the child's emotions. One of the most frequent side effects that we hear the most about with Ritalin is that the child becomes "zombie-like."

How Ritalin works is not fully known, but medical experts at universities conclude that Ritalin stimulates activity in parts of the brain that aids in concentration and impulse control, and raises the serotonin level in the brain.

But tryptophan, an amino acid which has no side effects whatsoever, raises the serotonin level of the brain naturally.

The traditional medical treatment for hyperactivity has been, and still is, the administration of behavior altering drugs like Ritalin, Cylert, or even in some cases drugs such as Atarax, Haladol, Elavil, Thorazine, Xanax, and Mellaril. These are the drugs that have been reported--how many others are used is not known.

When a child is kept on one of these controlled drugs, the cause is still there. In short, the medication may keep a lid on the undesirable behavior of the hyperactive child, but it does absolutely nothing to solve the basic problem in the child's body and brain.

Effect of Food Additives

Ben F. Feingold, M.D., of San Francisco, in 1975 wrote a book entitled *Why Your Child Is Hyperactive.* This book quickly caught on throughout the nation. Dr. Feingold believes hyperactivity is mainly due to artificial food coloring, artificial flavors, and natural salicylates. Though he notes that some children are also affected by other items such as dust, pets, pollens and odors, he does not believe that allergy is directly related to hyperactivity. Dr. Feingold is quick to point out that Ritalin and Cylert, the most commonly prescribed medications for hyperactivity, contain artificial colorings. All food additives must be considered potential allergic or toxic troublemakers for the hyperactive child.

In some cases, a child may have an allergic reaction to a specific chemical additive; again, the total load of the chemical additives contained in the child's diet and his medication may produce a toxic effect. If a certain food is definitely implicated as an unwanted cause of hyperactivity or hyperkinetic behavior, it should be eliminated from the child's diet for at least three months. The food elimination diet is an excellent way to find out what foods your child is allergic to. Two time Nobel Prize Laureate, Dr. Linus Pauling says a child must follow a dietary regime that is not deficient in the essential nutrients. This echoes the principle that "you are what you eat,"--and what you *don't* eat. Dr. Carl Pfeiffer, noted orthomolecular physician and past director of the Brain Bio-Center, postulates one of the major underlying causes of hyperactivity in children is a chemical imbalance in the child's biochemistry. Dr. Pfeiffer, feels parents should have children removed from sugar, food additives and caffeine, then find out what nutrient deficiencies they have occurring.

Dr. Jeffrey Bland has written an extremely important statement: "There is an exciting new development in the field of neuropharmacology that for the first time, diet may have an impact on brain neurochemistry; amino acids can actually influence regulatory substances that may ultimately and clinically cause changes in mood, mind, memory, and behavior."

Effectiveness of Amino Acids

Diet alone cannot supply children with optimum levels of nutrients needed by their unique biochemical and nutritional condition. Amino acids are used for hyperactive behavior to restore the disturbed biochemical homeostasis causing impaired functions in the child's brain. The amino acids literally feed the brain and restore the balance that nature intended.

Amino acids are the building blocks of proteins in the body. We cannot live without these proteins. Our children were not born with Ritalin in their brain, how can they have a Ritalin deficiency?

When a brain cell is stimulated, it releases a neurotransmitter that carries the message to the next cell. The neurotransmitter fills the cell, causing that cell to be stimulated. Then another messenger is released. All of this happens in the brain in a split second, allowing the message to travel quickly from one cell to the next along neuropathways. There are thousands of these pathways that carry messages to specialized areas of the brain.

This means all messages come in at once with equal velocity. The child's brain is like a telephone switching station on Christmas when everyone is trying to call at once, all you get are busy signals, and the messages do not reach the proper receptor site.

Neurotransmitters have the responsibility for behavior and learning, and a deficiency has a dramatic effect on children or adults ability to learn and function in an orderly manner. Most children who are hyperactive and A.D.D. are born with a shortage of neurotransmitters, which tends to run in families, mainly on the male side. HYPERACTIVITY and A.D.D. children do not manufacture the needed extra neurotransmitters.

Where do we get neurotransmitters from . . . from the amino acids, GABA, glycine, taurine, tyrosine, glutamine and tryptophan. Do children or adults get enough through diet? NO, NO and NO! Balanced amino acid doses in the right combination and formulas produce the needed neurotransmitters naturally. Using a stimulant medication to try to produce this, is like a shotgun gun going off in the child's brain.

We've seen the success of using amino acids over the past 10 years and happy, healthy children who are drug free. Amino acids restore the balance nature intended.

Allergic Conditions

Allergic condition means that something is wrong biochemically such as faulty absorption, depressed immune system, Candida yeast infection, weakened adrenal gland cortex or your child is not taking the needed supplements. Common symptoms include:

Tension headaches	Backaches
Itchy eyes, red eyeballs	Frequency and burning on
Anal itch	urination
Fluid behind ear drums	Anemia
Ringing in the ears	Sluggishness
Hearing loss	Depression
Cracks at corners of mouth	Restlessness
Hoarseness	Nervousness
Rapid heart beat	Tremor
Palpitations	Emotional outbursts
Belching	Destructive behavior
Heartburn	Anxiety, fear
Indigestion	Phobias, panic attacks
Stomach aches	Spacey feeling
Spastic colon	Memory loss
Hives	Inability to concentrate
Eczema	Irritable behavior before or
Muscle cramps	after meals

Vitamin And Nutritional Deficiencies

This controversy will go on for years to come: Pediatricians will tell their patients not to worry..."Just feed your child a well-balanced diet, and he will get everything he needs."

Simply feeding a high quality diet to a hyperactive child cannot be equated to high quality *and optimal nutrition*. There are many complex factors in digestion, absorption, and even the transportation of food that could be faulty. Optimum nutritional benefits depend on a multitude of factors; everything must function smoothly from the time the first bite is taken until the nutrient reaches the body cells. If an imbalance occurs from improper body functions, you will have an excess or deficiency of some sort. If the imbalance continues, the problem can go from a minor to a major disease.

Our food today does not have the nutritional value we need. The foods are contaminated by the polluted air, antibiotics, chemicals and insecticides that are all toxic and harmful. Unless you are with your child every minute, then you are not sure exactly what he consumes. Fast foods have now entered the schools along with candy, cookies and soft drinks, all of which contain an extremely high content of sugar and caffeine. How can you possibly feed your child a perfectly well-balanced diet, pediatricians tell you to, when the nutrient value of the food is *less than 50 percent*. The U.S. Agricultural Department states the food is colored to "look good", but the nutritional value is not there. American people believe in the fallacy that if they consume the number of calories in specific food groups, their dietary needs will be met. This, of course, should include getting the proper number of vitamins, amino acids and minerals. But instead of being in an optimally nourished state, the person is suboptimally nourished. The state of your nutrition is the state of your health. Further, the absence of disease does not necessarily mean the presence of wellness.

So why should our children be exempt? Nutritional deficiency disorders can and do occur, and in our own country we see malnutrition by overconsumption undernutrition. This simply means we eat too much of too little.

If a child has food allergies and their intake is restricted, diet becomes a bigger problem along with absorption. This is a major problem not only with hyperactive and A.D.D. children, but adults with high stress.

Symptoms of Amino Acid Deficiencies

- Chronic Fatigue
- Food / Chemical Allergies
- Recurrent Ear Infections
- Frequent Colds
- Mental - Emotional Problems
- Hyperactivity
- Depression
- Anxiety
- Frequent Headaches
- Insomnia
- Learning Disabilities
- Learning Disorders
- Immune Dysfunction
- Neurological Disorders
- Blood Sugar Disorders
- Arthritis

Informational pamphlet / MetaMatrix Medical Laboratory

The Treatment Of

Hyperactivity

By Orthomolecular Therapy

Parents often do not realize their children's need for amino acids because they do not realize how busy the human body is--even small ones. Consider these facts:

- Every second the bone marrow makes 2.5 million red blood cells;

- Every four days most of the lining of the gastro-intestinal tract and the blood platelets are replaced;

- Most of the white blood cells are replaced every 10 days;

- A human has the equivalent of a new skin every 24 days.

All of this continuous repair work requires amino acids, and the requirements are vastly increased by disease, inborn metabolic errors, allergies or anything that causes stress on the body. For example, children with brain damage, Down's syndrome, etc. need more amino acids than the average child. A child suffering the grief of losing a parent endures a terrific strain on his nervous system, and this uses up huge quantities of amino acids. The same is true for the grief of an adult and for depression. In fact, virtually all stress states require an increase in the supply of amino acids.

A neurotransmitter is the chemical language sent between brain cells in the human brain. Inhibitory amino acids of the brain that can affect and control this chemical language include tryptophan, taurine, GABA, and glycine. GABA, for example, as an inhibitory neurotranmsitter slows the anxiety-related messages sent between the parts of the brain.

The following is a list of amino acids and vitamins that are used in a special formula at The Pain and Stress Therapy Center in our treatment program for hyperactive children. These special formulas contain specific amounts needed by the child's brain to correct hyperactive behavior. The shotgun approach is never used. Giving a child mega doses of amino acids will do more harm than good. Our clinical results over the past ten years have shown children on this program have marked improvement. We have an 80 percent success rate with hyperactive children after they come off Ritalin.

TRYPTOPHAN (See Update)

Tryptophan, an essential amino acid, is necessary to maintain the body in protein balance. It has a variety of important roles in mental activity. Serotonin is a neurotransmitter, and one of the chemicals in the brain that helps control moods. To have enough serotonin you need enough tryptophan, which is essential in its formation. B6 (pyridoxine) is needed to form serotonin. Many hyperactive children have low serotonin, tryptophan and B6 levels. Tryptophan raises the low levels of blood serotonin. Supplements containing Tryptophan and B6 can correct some of the biochemical disorders related to aggression.

Studies done at the North-Nassau Mental Health Center in Mannasett, New York show that sufferers of obsessive-compulsive behavior evidenced signs of improvement following treatment with tryptophan and B6. An article published by the *American College of Nutrition* (June, 1987), showed specific doses of Tryptophan can replace Ritalin and

Cylert. One of the things Ritalin does is bring up the serotonin level in the child's brain, but it *forces* it up. Tryptophan brings up the serotonin level gently and normally. Tryptophan doses should be based on the child's hyperactivity, and no two children are alike--they are all biochemically individual. With orthomolecular treatment, results are positive and the reduction in hyperactivity in most cases is often dramatic. The child exhibits, among other qualities, a willingness to cooperate with his parents and teachers. These changes are seen in a majority of children who have previously failed to improve with the use of stimulant drugs or tranquilizers. The majority of children the author sees have been exposed to every form of treatment and most known tranquilizers and sedatives, with little or no success in controlling their hyperactivity.

GABA (Gamma Amino Butyric Acid)

The amino acid of the "eighties and nineties". We have been researching GABA at the Pain & Stress Therapy Center since 1984.

What GABA does is lower the excitatory level of the cell that is about to receive the incoming information. If the stress, panic, fear, etc., is prolonged, GABA's ability to block the messages is decreased, and finally the process by which the signals are rated for priority breaks down and the frontal cortex is literally bombarded with anxiety messages.

With the limbic system firing broadside fight-or flight signals at the frontal cortex, the subject's ability to reason is diminished. The effects now can include fear of dying, pounding heart, sweating, trembling, tightness, weakness, loss of control, disorientation--the list is endless. Research has shown that GABA can actually mimic the tranquilizing effect of Valium and Librium but without the heavy sedated effects of these drugs. This information was first released for publication in 1970 in the *Biochemical Basis of Neuropharmacology*. Since that time, numerous studies have been published showing the successful use of GABA with anxiety-prone individuals.

Research done has shown that a child who constantly experiences 'what-if'-type anxiety , or what is termed 'anticipatory fear,' has empty GABA receptors in the brain. This means that the brain can be bombarded with random firings of excitatory messages. It is the receptor site in the brain that prevents the reception of all the random firings so that the brain does not become overwhelmed. In *Lancet*, August 14, 1982, a research report about tranquilizers and GABA transmission clearly stated that GABA is a major inhibitory transmitter in the mammalian central nervous system and that the agents that raise the brain's GABA concentration possess a sedative anticonvulsant property.

GABA is used on a regular basis at the Pain & Stress Therapy Center with positive results. Dose amounts will vary. (I personally take GABA, and find benefits in the reduction of the effects of both daily stress and the tension in my neck and shoulders--which is where stress loves to attack children as well as adults.) This is pure GABA, not a mix of nutrients.

The anxiety and stress of a hyperactive child is stored in the limbic system (the emotional part) of the brain. Under prolonged periods of stress the limbic system releases the anxiety-related messages to fire at the cortex, or the "thinking part" of the brain; the child becomes overwhelmed, and the result is either hyper-aggressive or hyper-passive behavior. The child has no control over himself.

GABA is assuming an ever enlarging role as a major influence on drugs--in many cases replacing them. We have found GABA to work exceptionally well in combination with other amino acids with hyperactive children, both aggressive and passive.

TAURINE

Taurine is needed for normal development and health of the central nervous system. It has been shown to be important in controlling hyperactive or hyperkinetic movements. Taurine, after GABA, is the second most important inhibitory transmitter in the brain. Its inhibitory effect is one source of taurine's anticonvulsant and antianxiety properties. Taurine in the brain is usually associated with zinc or manganese. It is also present in the eye. Diminished vision may be an early warning sign of the need for taurine supplementation.

TYROSINE

Tyrosine is the first breakdown of phenylalanine in the liver. It is an amino acid that is helpful in overcoming depression. Clinical studies have shown that tyrosine controls medication-resistant depression.

In 1980, in the *American Journal of Psychiatry,* a study by Dr. Alan Gelenberg of the Department of Psychiatry at Harvard Medical School discussed the role of tyrosine in the control of anxiety and depression. Dr. Gelenberg postulated that the lack of available tyrosine results in deficiency of the hormone norepinephrine at a specific location in the brain, which in turn relates to mood problems, such as depression.

Tyrosine, because of its role in assisting the body to cope physiologically with stress and building the body's natural store of adrenalin, deserves to be called "the stress amino acid." Stress exhaustion needs tyrosine, which is converted to dopamine, norepinephrine, and epinephrine (adrenalin).

Tyrosine is needed during stress to continue coping with stress physiologically. We use tyrosine at the Pain & Stress

Therapy Center to aid young teens, as well as adults, with recurrent depression. Tyrosine is also helpful with smoking withdrawal symptoms.

GLYCINE

Carl Pfeiffer, M.D., Ph.D.'s studies demonstrate glycine is an important factor in psychiatric disorders. Dr. Pfeiffer's findings indicate that when glycine was administered to psychiatric patients suffering from manic-depression, even those who were previously unresponsive to drugs achieved a major improvement.

Glycine can be used in reducing aggression; it can also be used as a sugar substitute and mixed with other amino acids. It has a sweet taste and dissolves in water readily. Glycine is probably the third major inhibitory neurotransmitter of the brain.

MAGNESIUM

Magnesium is most always deficient in hyperactive or A.D.D. children. Magnesium is necessary for proper brain energy and is the first mineral depleted when anyone--child or adult--is under stress. Magnesium is a stress mineral and deficiency can lead to hyperactive or ADD behavior.

Sherry Rogers, M.D., has done years of extensive studies on the physical and mental symptoms of magnesium deficiency. In her book, *Tired or Toxic,* Dr. Rogers states magnesium has a quieting effect on the central nervous system. Dr. Rogers notes both children and adults who have apprehensiveness, irritability, confusion, noise sensitivity, constant eye twitching, nervousness, tremors, muscle spasms, jerking muscles, back and neck pain and some anxiety and fatigue have a magnesium deficiency. We have observed this in both adults and children with hyperactivity and anxiety. There are tests to determine magnesium deficiency, but Dr.

Rogers notes most of these tests do not give enough information.

Magnesium is linked to being very significant in sugar metabolism and proper utilization of carbohydrates to create energy rather than fats. Magnesium is so very important in your child's diet, especially if he has been displaying hyper behavior.

Magnesium can be taken in liquid form or capsule. The dose will depend on the child's weight, build, and the amount of stress and possible allergies, both food or airborne. Magnesium deficiency causes mast cells to release much more histamine. Histamine is the culprit responsible for much of the hayfever misery that so many people suffer from.

Magnesium quiets the central nervous system. When it is added to the hyperactives diet, calming effects are sometimes seen immediately. Most magnesium is found inside the cell where it activates enzymes necessary for the metabolism of carbohydrates and amino acids. It helps utilize the Vitamin B complex along with vitamin C and E and is associated with the regulation of body temperature.

CALCIUM

A calcium deficiency may also induce hyperactivity. The low calcium child may be irritable, sleep disturbed, angry, and inattentive. Edginess disappears and calm prevails when the calcium needs are met. The first sign of a calcium deficiency is a nervous stomach, cramps, and tingling in the arms and legs. Calcium is a strong countering agent against lead; children with inadequate calcium in their diets appear to be more likely to get lead intoxication.

A child who is found to be food sensitive to dairy products is not likely to be receiving proper amounts of dietary calcium or tryptophan. In at least 50 percent of the children we test for food sensitivities, we find them to have a sensitivity to dairy products. Yet diary products are a major food source of tryptophan. So if the child's diet is restricted from all dairy products, he should be given these vital nutrients in supplements form.

One should note that bananas are extremely high in tryptophan and hence serotonin; they are very good for children.

ZINC

Zinc controls protein synthesis in every cell of the body and is thus associated with burn and wound healing, carbohydrate digestion, and organ growth development. Zinc deficiency is a factor involved in fatigue, susceptibility to infection, decreased appetite, alertness, loss of taste, and prolonged wound healing. Important constituents in the body activity involve zinc, chromium, and magnesium as well as the hormone insulin. Insulin is essential for the regulation of blood sugar levels.

B VITAMINS

Several years ago, Dr. Marvin Brend found first signs of Vitamin B deficiency in the psychological category with symptoms such as fear, depression, temper tantrums, anxiety, mood swings, inability to concentrate, withdrawal, listlessness, and a general feeling of being tired. Dr. Brend suggested that the weakening effects of B Vitamin deficiency occur well before a person actually displays an acute vitamin deficiency sign.

Doctors Cschamberger and Longsdale, at Cleveland Clinic, further confirmed that children with behavior disorders were found to have chronic marginal B deficiencies. The signs of deficiencies include aggressive personality changes, sleep problems, reoccurring bad dreams and heightened anxiety. The researchers were able to associate these symptoms with the consumption of diets rich in "empty" calories, meaning foods high in sugar and fat but low in vitamins and minerals. Many of the snack conveniences today, fall into this category of empty calories.

Parents must constantly be aware of how many of these high sugar empty calorie snacks their child consumes daily, for this helps determine the behavioral pattern. Marginal vitamin deficiency signs and symptoms are associated with conditions that are often missed by many physicians because they are nutrient related, and many physicians receive little if any education on nutrition and vitamins while in medical school. As a result, they are simply not aware of this relationship. Some of the first signs of vitamin deficiencies include: intestinal problems of unknown origin, muscle pain, sleep disturbances, headaches, emotional problems, constant fatigue and lack of energy. These symptoms may be significantly improved by a proper nutrient supplementation program. There could still be conditions of emotional or mental disturbance that are not related to nutrient deficiencies and could require behavior therapy. But it is most important for a parents to recognize the physical and emotional signs and symptoms of vitamin deficiencies in their child and take appropriate action before those deficiencies show in a much broader range of symptoms.

A nutrient is different from a drug; a nutrient is a food substance that in most cases supplies either the energy or the molecular building blocks the body requires. There are some nutrients that, when administered in their pure form or simply ingested in food, can act like drugs. They give rise to important changes in the chemical composition of structures in the brain. These changes can modify brain function, particularly in people with certain metabolic or neurologic diseases.

NIACINAMIDE (B3)

Niacinamide is another vitamin that offers help for the hyperactive child. Especially encouraging in reports of the use of this vitamin is the fact that it has a settling influence on a distractable child. The effect is much different from that of Ritalin dosage; the quieting effect on the nervous system is much better. Nor does niacinamide cause the flush and rapid heart beat that occurs with pure niacin.

CALCIUM PANTOPHENATE (B5)

Calcium pantophenate is another used to help modulate the behavior of a hyperactive child. When B5 is added in doses of 15 to 50 mg with Ester C and niacinamide, results have been positive in the treatment of hyperactive children with aggressive behavior. This particular nutrient supports the adrenal system of the child under heavy stress, anxiety, and depression. B5 is an anti-allergic.

Never use more than 50 mg without the directions of a healthcare professional.

PYRIDOXINE (B6)

This is one of the most important nutrients. B6 is one of the greatest fighters against hyperactivity. It calms the hyperactive child in much the same way as Vitamin B. Vitamin B6 and tryptophan supplements can correct some biochemical disorders related to aggression. B6 is the most important vitamin for amino acid metabolism because it is the cofactor for the enzymes called transamines, which metabolize amino acids. Riboflavin (B2) and Niacin (B3) are the next most important vitamins in amino acid metabolism. B6 must be used with amino acids.

VITAMIN C OR ESTERIFIED C

Vitamin C is most important in the treatment of hyperactivity. The most recent clinical studies in 1987 established

Ester C Polyascorbate as totally neutral; it is proven four times more bioavailable than ordinary Vitamin C. Ester C is a unique complex mixture with a different molecular personality. This means that Ester C is the most available form of Vitamin C to the tissues of the body. It is also in your system within 20 minutes after ingesting and 24 hours later, working long after even timed-released forms of Vitamin C have been excreted from the body. Children, as well as adults need Vitamin C daily. Ester C has been extremely effective in our program, and it does not cause diarrhea or gastrointestinal upsets that can happen with regular ascorbic acid, Vitamin C. Ester C has a neutral pH of 7.0. Dr. Jeffrey Bland, nutritional biochemist and foremost authority today in nutritional therapy / medicine recommends a range of 300 to 1000 mg of Ester C for children daily. At The Pain & Stress Center, we include the Ester C in every child's program for hyperactivity. Ester C is available in a pediatric dose of 275 or 550 mg. We have had excellent response from most children using it. Ester C given on a daily basis is the most inexpensive nutritional insurance policy you will ever find, with positive, long-term beneficial effects on your child's health.

VITAMIN E

Vitamin E is absolutely essential to normal function of every cell in the body. It is being used in the treatment of hyperactive children with positive results.

Wilfrid Shute, M.D., in his book *Health Preserver*, in defining the versatility of Vitamin E, established that hyperactive children have a deficiency of Vitamin E. Dr. Shute states he has obtained remarkable results with Vitamin E, not only in hyperactivity but also in learning disabilities and attention deficit disorder. Dr. Shute says that Vitamin E improves the child's ability to learn through a defective or damaged sensory channel. While it does not change the basic personality of the child, it does enhance his ability to learn, an improvement which occurs slowly but steadily.

Vitamin E would be helpful in both aggressive or passive hyperactivity. Since it is required for normal cell functioning, Dr. Shute feels it should be kept in a child's - -and even in adult's--daily regimen; 400 I.U. is recommended for a child under 10.

A recent patient at our clinic was a 14 year old girl who was withdrawn and anxious and had numerous skin problems. With the daily use of 800 I.U. of Vitamin E, in three weeks her skin began to clear and her confidence improved. If a child feels different or feels rejected from others because he is different in some way, behavior problems can occur, especially passive hyperactivity. Nutritional deficiencies have to be addressed, especially children's.

L-GLUTAMINE

Tests have shown that glutamic acid, a "non-essential" amino acid, improves intelligence, speeds the healing of ulcers, gives a "lift" from fatigue, and helps control alcoholism, schizophrenia, and the craving for sweets. The problem is that in order to get more of this amino acid into the brain where it becomes a high-energy brain fuel, we have to use a little nutritional ingenuity.

Feeding moderate amounts of *L-glutamine* produces marked elevation of glutamic acid in the brain. The relationship of glutamic acid to glucose goes beyond their brain-fuel interrelationship. Glutamic acid restores hypoglycemic patients in insulin coma to consciousness at a lower blood sugar level than when glucose alone is used. The brain can store only a small reserve of glucose; therefore, it is very dependent on the second-to-second supply of blood sugar. This explains the dizziness and other nervous symptoms in hypoglycemics.

Glutamic acid is the only other compound used for energy by the brain; the gray matter contains a special enzyme to convert glutamic acid into a compound that regulates brain cell activity. Glutamic acid is used in a special high energy reaction that bypasses the normal energy producing chemistry of the citric acid cycle. Thus, a shortage of L- glutamine in the diet, or glutamic acid in the brain, results in brain damage due to excess ammonia or a brain that can never "get into high gear."

Dr. Roger Williams at the Clayton Foundation, University of Texas at Austin in his many years of research, established the importance of the amino acid, glutamine in brain function. Glutamine is known as the M & C amino acid, memory and concentration. Seventy five percent of hyperactive and A.D.D. children tested using serum plasma were found to have a low level of glutamine.

Dr. C. Frederiscks has seen an increase in the IQ's of children given glutamine. When glutamine was given daily, impressive improvements were seen in the child's ability to learn, to retain and to recall.

A major part of my orthomolecular program for hyperactive and A.D.H.D children is adding glutamine in supplement form. Glutamine is one of the amino acids that create the needed neurotransmitters in the brain which enhances learning and memory. Often hyperactive and A.D.D. children that are tested have low neurotransmitter levels, especially glutamine. Start with 500 mg of glutamine and gradually increase until the optimal dose is obtained for your child. The dosage depends on your child's weight, activity and concentration level. The total maximum recommended glutamine dosage is 3000 mg per day. When the child is able to concentrate and learn you have reached his optimum dosage.

Research has discovered that L-glutamine protects bacteria cells against poisoning by alcohol, and in experimentation on laboratory rats it stopped their craving for alcohol. This property has been studied carefully, and compared with the effects of other amino acids, but L- glutamine consistently decreased alcohol consumption.

The brain must be nourished to function properly; whatever the brain tells the body to do, the body does. Everything starts with the brain and ends in the brain. As I mentioned before, the composition and the function of the brain can be altered by the amino acids, tryptophan, tyrosine, and GABA. These amino acids are precursors in the brain, and ultimately affect everyone's behavior.

The most exciting area of amino acid research is the study of brain metabolism. Amino acids therapies are making a great impact on general medicine, and in the field of psychiatry.

Dr. Alexander Brawley, Director of MetaMatrix Laboratories, a licensed clinical lab specializing in amino acid and vitamins levels states that specific amino acids are necessary for proper neurological functioning. Subtle deficiencies of these can affect mental and emotional stability. Supplementation of specific amino acids is useful in treating hyperactivity, depression, anxiety, headaches, P.M.S., mental confusion, poor memory, and concentration.

Amino acids serve as an important anti-inflammatory substance that helps control sensitivity reactions and the body's natural response system. Many children and adults with food allergies report improved tolerance of food with amino acid supplementation.

Dr. William Walsh is an authority on the diagnosis and treatment of biochemical imbalances that result in behavioral disorders, including violent behavior. He has developed a treatment program to control chemical imbalances with the late Dr. Carl Pfeiffer. The program consists of carefully controlled combinations of vitamins, minerals, and amino acids. His results were overwhelmly positive.

Does Dr. Walsh advocate Ritalin? No. Is Ritalin the answer? No. Does Dr. Rapp, the world's foremost authority in pediatric allergy and immunology, advocate Ritalin? No. Would I give Ritalin to my child? No.

Food Allergy Screening

Recent interest in the food allergy problem has risen from a expanding recognition in the medical literature of the pervasive nature of food sensitivity. It has been estimated that 60% of the U.S. population suffers some form of food allergy that can either cause or complicate a health problem. The symptoms associated with an adverse food reaction are extraordinarily diverse. (See page 12 - 13 for symptoms.)

There are two major types of food reactions:
1. Immediate 2. Delayed.

Immediate Food Reactions

Food reactions which occur within 3 hours after eating are called immediate. Generally they are assumed to be caused by high IgE antibody levels present in the blood that produce an immediate allergic reaction. This would be the "classic" allergy reaction many people are familiar with. Obvious reactions such as a rash or headache after eating or drinking an offending food.

Delayed Food Reactions

A delayed reaction generally occurs hours or up to 3 days after consuming the offending food. Sometimes you may eat a food for several days, then develop a reaction to it. Delayed reactions are usually more difficult to recognize, and are often called hidden food allergies.

The immune response to delayed food reactions is more complex and less defined than in the immediate type reaction. In most cases delayed reactions involve other antibodies such as IgG, IgM, and IgA. These combine with the food particles in the blood, forming complexes that evidently cause inflammatory reactions in tissues.

Special Consideration Of

Circumstances

Children and Grief

One of the most difficult problems for parents is helping a child through the crisis of death of a parent or grandparent or even another child he is very close to.

Children's feelings and perceptions are often overlooked. Grief is a deeply human emotion, as normal as laughing, playing, crying or sleeping. Grief is a way of saying, "I miss you, and I do not understand where you are ... or where you have gone." When you avoid a child's reaction, you magnify his fears and replace reality with fantasy or psychological defenses.

Often the surviving parent is caught up with his or her grief and makes the mistake of not addressing the child's needs. The child will begin to act out his fears, depression, anxiety, and most of all, the uncertainty of being left alone-- of being abandoned. This behavior can be interpreted as hyperactivity though it is simply the result of the child's frustration.

If your family has lost a loved one, take this into consideration *before* someone tells you your child is hyperactive. Many times we have had parents say, "Since his father died, I haven't been able to reach him." This child is in need of behavior therapy. If he does not receive proper counseling, his hostility will continue to grow and come out in physical form such as picking on other children, striking at their surviving parent, breaking things, etc.

A special note here: Before the age of twelve, it is very hard for a child to understand death. Taking them to funerals where people are grieving, or having them kiss the loved one "good-bye" in most cases can have a totally negative effect. We have seen many adults who were still haunted by the memory of having to kiss a dead person good-bye. The mental state of a child is so delicate that all of these things must be taken into consideration.

Children and Divorce

If you are in the process of, or have recently received, a divorce, your children will need time to adjust to this major transitional change in their life. A recent study presented to the American Association for Marriage and Family Therapy, October, 1988, by the Society for Research in Adolescence, showed divorce and remarriage are hardest on children ages 9 to 15. The study was conducted with 210 families. It is important to recognize that children in this age group are struggling to establish independence, self- esteem, and sexual identity.

Parents are role models for their children, and when one is gone, a child under ten does not understand. Your child needs reassurance that you too will not go away. He also needs time to express his feelings, fears, anxiety, and guilt. He may feel he did something wrong--even that he or she was the cause of the divorce. Only through helping him understand will these feelings go away. Do not take your child for granted, thinking that he will get over it in due time. Unless you talk to your child, the only other information he gets is from other children, which is not a reliable source.

Divorce is loss, separation, and there will be a certain amount of grief on the part of the child as well as the parent. The reaction of the child to this loss may be similar to a loss through death--disruptive behavior, lashing out at everyone, and anger. Some parents say that their child becomes unmanageable since their divorce, and that his teachers are complaining about his behavior.

Preventive Measures

One essential preventive measure which a parent should take even before the divorce, separation, or an impending death, is inform school officials. By understanding the reason for a child's behavior they can become an important support system for the child.

My own experience can serve as an example in this situation. When I was a very small child, I lost my father. I had already been through a major trauma from a burn received at 14 months of age. Now I had to cope with this loss, and I could not understand why it happened. There were three other children in the house and my mother worked full- time, so there was very little time for me to express all of my thoughts and feelings which were many. Mother simply did not have the time--and perhaps not the awareness-to see what I was experiencing. These bewildered feelings stayed locked inside me for a long time.

When I was eight, my mother packed up all our belongings, and without explanation, we left Cleveland, Ohio by train for Seattle, Washington. It was not until we were one day out of Seattle that my mother sat me down, and told me, she planned to remarry. I felt betrayed, lonely, and very angry. My behavior took on passive hyperactivity. I withdrew, talked very little, and did not understand all that had happened. My teachers began to complain to my mother about my withdrawal. My mother confronted me with my behavior. I was only able to give her bits and pieces of explanation but promised to do better. Through the understanding and gentleness of a very concerned nun, I was able to resolve some of my feelings, and my behavior improved.

But it was not until my thirties that I was able to sort out some of the unresolved anxiety and anger.

A frequent reaction to divorce is for the child to compete with the new parent for the attention of the natural parent, and the resulting conflict can cause stress and then depression. A child must be prepared when a parent remarries and only when the youngster's acceptance is sure should the wedding take place. This procedure will ensure that the family unit remains close.

If your child is going through this type of stress, it is a perfect time to use tryptophan for both sleep problems and depression, and GABA for anxiety, or in combination. This is a crucial time for both you and your child.

Never tell your children what they will need to unlearn at a later time. At a time of crisis, the whole family suffers; this calls for understanding, communication, trust, and truth between parents and children.

Children in times of stress need more neurotransmitters. The immune system is totally depleted, and they tend to turn to junk food and sweets for satisfaction. You should make sure they receive proper supplementation to help them in times of crisis.

Please see Tryptophan Update.

Behavior Characteristics of

Hyperactive and A.D.D.

Children

The hyperactive A.D.D. child displays a multitude of behavior characteristics. Most of these are the inability of the central nervous system to effectively modulate motor activity.

A significant factor about hyperactivity is that it really affects less than thirty percent of the individuals with attention deficit disorder. This is an extremely interesting point, since for many years everyone with attention deficit syndrome was referred to as hyperactive. The range of hyperactivity is from minor fidgetiness or finger tapping to the more overt behavior of hyperkinesis, when the child is in perpetual motion from dawn to dark.

Hyperactive children usually have restless sleep cycles and short sleep patterns. The sleep pattern is affected by a low serotonin level.

Mary Coleman, M.D., Ph.D. found all hyperactive children have a serotonin level which varied by her study. A proper combination of tryptophan and B6 will bring this level into balance, and the child's symptoms would diminish. The dosage of course, would depend on the child's age, weight, and the degree of hyperactivity. As stated before, when you correct nutrient deficiencies and the brain is fed properly, the child's behavior changes accordingly.

One of the behaviors most often mistaken for A.D.D. is chronic anxiety. Here a child can display both aggressive and passive behavior. They cling to their parents and fear any new situations, or constantly argue. Low self esteem, frustration and dependency are part of the hyper A.D.D. child's behavior.

The child wants help and does not understand why he behaves the way he does. If he is taking Ritalin, he becomes more withdrawn and will not verbalize his feelings. Young children don't know how to say, "Please help." But they will say, "Please don't make me take Ritalin anymore."

These were the words of a little boy named Scott in 1984 when his mother brought him to my office to evaluate his aggressive behavior. The question in my mind was why Ritalin, a powerful stimulant. My search began for the proper nutrients that affect brain chemistry, and would help children without being harmful. Scott's problem was specific amino acids and allergic reactions to what his mother thought was the best thing she could give him, milk. The milk was eliminated from Scott's diet and his behavior improved remarkably.

Hyperactivity or Allergic Reactions

In 1988 when I wrote the first edition of *Control Hyperactivity* I briefly mentioned food allergies and chemical sensitivities as a cause of hyperactivity and A.D.D. Since that time I have had the opportunity to work with Dr. Doris Rapp, who I and millions of others, consider the world's foremost authority in this field. For her contributions I hope and pray Dr. Rapp is given a Nobel prize. She truly deserves it.

Through her books, tapes, lectures and personal consults I have come to realize thousands of children are misdiagnosed because the physician is not aware of what he is treating. Every pediatrician in this country should read, *Is This Your Child?* And I encourage every parent to make this investment in their child's health.

The following are behavioral indications of children who may have an unrecognized sensitivity to food, dust, molds, pollens, or chemicals:

- One day (or hour) learns well but the next day (or hour) he can't
- Appears unable to learn or behave most of the time
- Suffers from recurrent headaches, leg aches, muscle spasms, digestive complaints or bedwetting
- Seems unable to function consistently well in school
- Behavior and personality swings between Dr. Jekyll and Mr. Hyde
- Too active or too tired

If any of these symptoms fit your child, then you should certainly look in the direction of the problem area, and begin to correct it as soon as possible. There is a wide range of illnesses, but if the problems can be recognized early in the infant or toddler stage, many emotional, learning and health problems that interfere with a child's ability to reach full potential can be prevented.

Most parents never suspect that their children's or their own medical or emotional complaints can be due to an environmental illness. There are a multitude of warning signs along the way, but most parents don't pay any attention until notes start coming home from school or the child is in the second or third grade and doing poorly.

Parents should be aware of behavior at an early age. A baby who falls out the crib at an early age, walks at eight months, has one ear infection after another with a lot of congestion and formula changes, you should suspect a possible allergy connection. Be aware of toddlers who have constant temper tantrums, classical nose allergies, aches in the legs, stomach aches and gas. By the time they start school, they can't sit still, are irritable, aggressive, bite, punch, and kick parents as well as other children. They may cough when they laugh or run or exercise when exposed to cold air and cold drinks. On damp days, they start wheezing and you're sure they are getting asthma.

Some children become fatigued, withdrawn, irritable, and pull away if you try to touch them. When some children have a reaction, they may cringe and hide somewhere in a dark corner. Some are depressed and suicidal after eating certain foods or being exposed to pollens, molds, dust or chemical odors. Many have short fuses and will explode with anger and rage for no apparent reason. They fear rejection and withdraw from relationships.

Handwriting is a tell tale way to follow the hyperactive child's behavior--they may go from large to small dots. Certain children develop characteristic appearances when they are having a reaction. They include puffy bags under the eyes, red ears, dark blue, black or red eye circles, nose rubbing, wiggly legs, spaced out look, demon look. These signs reflect the behavioral patterns of the allergic tension fatigue syndrome. Other typical allergic reactions such as asthma, hayfever, eczema or hives along with muscle aches and spasms, headaches, leg aches, irritability, fatigue, depression, belligerence, temper tantrum, disturbed sleep, bedwetting, digestive upset and learning difficulties. Some children do not have typical allergic responses, only the later complaints, which are not usually recognized by allergists and physicians as being related to allergies.

Many of these varying clusters of problems are indeed caused by an allergic reaction to different foods, chemicals, dust, pollen and molds. Dr. Doris Rapp believes allergies can strike anywhere on or in the body, and affect the emotions. She does not believe allergies are just limited to hives, hayfever and asthma because of an allergic reaction. Some also have wild mood swings and the inability to learn for the same reason.

Dr. Rapp's views are shared by over 3,000 physicians and therapists who practice environmental and orthomolecular medicine. They are convinced that many behavioral, emotional and physical problems, that are not conventionally accepted as being due to allergy, can readily be caused by sensitivity to different factors in the environment or diet.

Many doctors think allergies affect 10 to 15 percent of the population, but I believe this kind of illness is much more common. In some schools there are estimated 25 percent of children on Ritalin. And if you ask teachers who have been teaching for twenty or thirty years, they will tell you there is no comparison to how children were before and how they are now. "The problems don't end with childhood," says Dr. Rapp. "The disease inside little bodies continues and you eventually have an irritable, repressed, and fatigued adult, who doesn't live up to his or her potential, can't form a good relationship with the opposite sex, or who can't hold a job."

Dr. Rapp questions how many general practitioners, psychiatrists, pediatricians, neurologists, psychologists, teachers, or parents are *not* aware that food pollens, molds, dust, mites, pets, and chemical pollution are clearly environmental factors. Any of these can cause some children to become hyperactive, inattentive and impulsive. If environmental factors are not considered, many children can be needlessly placed on Ritalin.

Those factors are found anywhere--home, school, inside or outside. There could be a sensitivity to a pet, a carpet cleaning chemical or the synthetic carpet itself, to mouthwash, to the toothpaste with red dye and sugar, to the teachers perfume. All are possibilities. You need to play detective.

In many school districts, the use of ventilation systems is reduced to cut heating or cooling bills. The resultant poor air circulation can affect sensitive children who may then react to chemicals and disinfectants in the bathrooms, on the desktops, the floors, in the gym or in the cafeteria. Children will become limp or hyperactive from the sprays used on their desks in the classroom. When the children go outside, instead of fresh air, they may encounter air laden with pesticides, fungicides or herbicides and all sorts of things. Some schools allow smoking in the bathrooms. A sensitive youngster can enter a lavatory, encounter a barrage of odors and chemicals, and exit in an altered state, unable to write or concentrate in class.

You may have to go to school, as some parents do, and literally see, smell and touch your child's environment. Walk into the gym. Do you smell fresh floor wax? You may have to visit the principal and request a moratorium on floor wax for a couple of weeks and see if there are any changes. In cooperation with school authorities some parents have installed air purifiers to clean up the air in their children's classrooms. The purifier helps to remove dust, molds and chemicals. Affected children often improve. Entire classrooms often experience fewer infections.

When you figure out the cause, you can do something about it. But if parents don't take the time, nobody else will. Read as much as possible on the allergy behavior connection and, if possible bring the affected child to a specialist in environmental medicine. These practitioners help parents remove the nails from the shoe and don't just put ointment on the sore. Parents are taught how to recognize and remove the causes of their children's illness in preference to treating the effects with drugs.

Educated parents should no longer feel helpless or guilty. You quickly learn to recognize why your child suddenly becomes ill or acts inappropriately. Once you see improvement after changes are made in the diet, at home or school environments, you can make the types of decisions which promote long-term wellness rather than chronic illness within the family.

When parents combine the nutritional approach with the possible allergy related problems, they give their children a chance to heal naturally, an approach they will use throughout life. Drug free!

Amino Acids Are Vital

The body requires daily at least 20 times as much in amino acid intake as it does in vitamins, and about four times as much as the minerals. This requirement has to be in the form of free amino acids for best results, not protein in undigested lumps. When we have an efficient digestive function, the breakdown of protein can occur, releasing an adequate supply of free form amino acids.

The scope and use of the proper amino acids in therapy can seem to be enormous. If all of the amino acids in their free form, are not present in adequate amounts, there will be an imbalance in the neurotransmitter function and a hyperactive / A.D.D. behavior will result. The energy of the brain is dependent on certain amino acids.

Common Symptoms
Of Food Allergies

PHYSICAL SYMPTOMS:

Skin:

Hives, rash, eczema, dermatitis, pallor.

Head:

Insomnia, faintness, headaches, dizziness, feeling of fullness in the head, excessive drowsiness or sleepiness soon after eating.

Eyes, Ears, Nose, and Throat: Stuffy nose, runny nose, excessive mucous formation, post nasal drip, watery eyes, earache, fullness of ears, fluid in the middle, hearing loss, recurrent ear infections, itching ear, ear drainage, sore throats, chronic cough, gagging, canker sores, itching of the roof of the mouth, recurrent sinusitis.

Heart and Lungs: Increased heart rate, asthma, palpitations, congestion in the chest, arrythmias, tachycardia.

Gastrointestinal: Nausea, vomiting, diarrhea, constipation, bloating after meals, belching, colitis, flatulence (passing gas), feeling of fullness in the stomach long after finishing a meal, abdominal pains or cramps.

Other Symptoms: Chronic fatigue, weakness, muscle aches and pains, joint aches and pains, arthritis, swelling of the hands, feet or ankles, urinary tract symptoms such as frequency of urination or urgency, vaginal itching, vaginal discharge, hunger, "binge" or "spree" eating.

PSYCHOLOGICAL SYMPTOMS:

Anxiety, "panic" attacks, depression, crying jags, aggressive behavior, irritability, mental dullness, mental lethargy, confusion, excessive daydreaming, hyperactivity, restlessness, learning disabilities, poor work habits, slurred speech, stuttering, inability to concentrate, indifference.

Various Foods Known To Cause Allergy

Almond	Cranberry	Peppers (red or green)
Apple	Cucumber	Persimmon
Apricot	Currant	Pineapple
Arrowroot	Eggs	Plum
Artichoke	Eggplant	Pork
Asparagus	Fig	Potato, white
Banana	Fish, all types	Prunes
Beans	Garlic	Pumpkin
Beef	Ginger	Rhubarb
Beet	Gooseberry	Rice
Blueberry	Grape	Sassafras
Brazil nut	Leek	Scallop
Broccoli	Lentils	Seafoods
Brussels sprouts	Lettuce	Shrimp
Buckwheat	Mango	Soy products
Cabbage	Melons	Spices
Carrot	Milk	Spinach
Cashew	Mushrooms	Squash
Cauliflower	Mustard	Strawberries
Celery	Nuts	Sweet potato
Cherry	Oats	Sugar
Chicken	Okra	Tapioca
Chocolate	Olives	Tomatoes
Citrus fruits	Onions	Turkey
Clam	Oranges	Turnip
Cloves	Oyster	Vanilla
Cocoa	Peach	Walnuts
Coconut	Peas	Wheat
Coffee	Peanuts	Wintergreen
Corn	Pecans	Yeast

Signs And Symptoms of Cow's Milk Allergy

GASTROINTESTINAL
Abdominal pain
Abdominal distention
Colic in infants
Colitis (inflammation of colon)
Constipation Stomachache
Diarrhea
Gas
Heartburn
Indigestion
Intestinal obstruction in infants
Malabsorption
Mouth ulcers
Peptic ulcers
Poor appetite
Rectal bleeding
Vomiting

MISCELLANEOUS
Red eyes due to allergy
Anaphylaxis
Anemia
Arthritis-like symptoms
Bad breath
Bedwetting
Behavior disorders
Cardiac irregulatities
Right heart failure
Cystitis
Excessive sweating
Failure to thrive
Fatigue
"Growing pains"
Headache
Heart disease

Hyperactivity
Irritability
Lassitude
Vaginal discharge
Migraine
Musculoskeletal discomfort
Nephrotic syndrome
Paleness
Pallor
Polyarthritis
Tension
Thrombocytopenia

RESPIRATORY
Asthma
Bronchitis
Cough
Croup
Earache
Frequent colds
Hair loss
Nasal congestion
Nose bleeds
Recurrent pneumonia
Postnasal drip
Runny nose
Sinusitis
Sore throat
Stuffy nose
Wheezing

SKIN /
DERMATOLOGICAL
Acne
Swollen lips
Dark circles around eyes
Eczema
Hives

Warning Signs Of Inadequate Nutrition

ORGAN SYSTEM	PHYSICAL SIGNS	NUTRIENT DEFICIENCY
Neck	Goiter	Iodine
Teeth	Dental cavities	Fluoride
	Mottled enamel	Excessive Fluoride
	Cavities	Vitamin C
		Phosphorus
	Malposition	Protein-calorie
Tongue	Red, painful, sore	B6 (Pyridoxine)
		Folic Acid
	Swollen	Iron
	Purple in color	Riboflavin
	Scarlet, raw	Niacin

Mouth	Sore; cracked and chapped lips	Riboflavin
Face	Brown, patchy pigmentatin of cheeks, parotid enlargement, "moon" face	Protein-calorie
Lips	Inflammation of the mucus membranes of the lips	Riboflavin
Nose	White and black heads along border of nose and cheeks	B6 (Pyridoxine)
Gums	Hypertrophy or overgrowth of gums Inflammation of gums	Vitamin C Vitamin A Niacin Riboflavin
Eyes	Extreme sensitivity to light, poor twilight vision, loss of shine, bright and moist appearance, loss of light reflex, decreased tears, softening of cornea	Vitamin A
	Inside of eye lid is pale	Iron or Folate
	Tissue at external angles of both eyes is moist and red	Riboflavin
Nails	Ridging, brittle, easily broken, flattened, spoon-shaped, thin, lusterless	Iron

Hair	Becomes dull, fine, brittle, straight Becomes red in Blacks, then lighter in color; may be "bleached" in Whites, is easily and painlessly pluckable, outer one-third of eyebrow may be sparse in hypothyroidism (cretinism, iodine deficiency, or other causes)	Protein-calorie
Skin	Dryness of skin, follicular hyperkaeratosis ("gooseflesh," "sharkskin," "sandpaper skin,") acne lesions	Vitamin A
	Red spots which produce "pink-halo" effects around coiled hair follicles, purple bruises in skin due to capillary fragility, bleeds into joints, cortical hemorhages of bone visisble on x-ray	Vitamin C
	Hemorrhages in skin, gastrointestinal hemorrhages	Vitamin K
	Pallor, jaundice	Vitamin B12
	Pallor	Iron
	Redness of the skin occurring in patches of variable size and shape early, then vascularization, crusting, shedding. Increased pigmentation, thickened, inelastic, fissures in skin, especially in skin exposed to sun, becoming scaley, dry pigmentation of the cheek and above the eye	Niacin

System	Signs/Symptoms	Nutrient
Skeletal	Osteoporosis (in association with low protein intake and floride deficiency)	Calcium
	Growth part of bone is enlarged, painless. "Beading" of ribs, delayed fusion of cranial fontanelles, bowed legs, deformities of thorax (such as pigeon breast), osteomalacia (adults)	Vitamin D
	Hematoma in bone, enlargement of the growth part of bones, painless	Vitamin C
Muscular	Loss of tone	Vitamin D
	Muscle wasting, weakness, fatigue, inactivity; loss of subcutaneous fat	Protein-calorie
	Accumulation of blood within muscles	Vitamin C
	Calf muscle tenderness, weakness	Thiamine
Central Nervous System (CNS)	Apathy, irritability, psychomotor changes	Protein
	Psychotic behavior (dementia)	Niacin
	Peripheral neuropathy, symmetrical sensory and motor deficits, especially in lower extremities, drug-resistant	B6 (Pyridoxine)

CNS (continued)	convulsions (infants), dementia, forgetfulness	
	Lack of reflexes, loss of position and vibratory senses, tingling of skin	Vitamin B12
	Tremors, convulsions, behavioral disturbances	Magnesium
Liver	Fatty infiltration of liver	Protein-calorie
Gastrointestinal	Anorexia, flatulence, diarrhea	Vitamin B12
	Anorexia	Zinc
	Diarrhea	Niacin, Protein-calorie
Cardiovascular	Rapid heartbeat, congestive heart failure, heart enlargement, electro-cardiographic changes	Thiamine

The Bewildering World of

Childhood

Today's world surrounds our children with stressors and uncertainties, fears and anxieties which you and I never faced. The fifties and sixties certainly had their own wars and uncertainties, but consider the child of today. Use your own imagination for just a minute.

What would it be like if you were just seven? A seven year old is faced with the possibility of nuclear war, death and dying, and the end of the world; they are aware of the homeless who live in the streets, and they are surrounded by a sea of drugs offered to them from every direction with the echo, "Just say NO." This child of seven sees his own parents using drugs, drinking and driving, and he is constantly frightened by the possibility of physical abuse.

I believe that some hyperactive behavior comes from fear, uncertainty, and not knowing who to trust or where to turn. I feel that as parents we must be more believable, while making sure that we listen to what the small voice is trying to say.

As a parent, if you feel down deep that your child's behavior is unrealistic and beyond what you can help him with, do not hesitate to find a behavior therapist who has empathetic understanding.

Carl Rogers, in his book, *A Way Of Being,* states, "Empathetic understanding is a way of being with another person. It means entering the private perceptual world of another and becoming thoroughly at home in it."

Empathetic understanding means you can walk the same path . . . and understand their soft crying out.

Tryptophan Update

In November, 1989, the F.D.A. ordered the amino acid tryptophan removed from the public. As of February, 1994 they still have not released it! Tryptophan was used by millions of people for over 40 years. No significant problems were noted until 1988. Then a rare condition known as E.M.S. (Eosinophilia Myalgia Syndrome) surfaced and was traced to one contaminated batch of tryptophan. The problem occurred in the manufacturing phase in tryptophan made by Showa Denko. Showa Denko, a Japanese firm, corrected the error, but the F.D.A. would not release tryptophan to the millions of adults and children who desperately need it. Tryptophan has been cleared by the C.D.C. (Centers for Disease Control) for release. For many without tryptophan, they would have to turn to toxic, addictive drugs.

The F.D.A. has been given documented studies done with pure pharmaceutical grade tryptophan and the contaminated batch tryptophan. Utilizing the pure tryptophan produced NO problems, but problems existed with the contaminated tryptophan. Tryptophan is safe! This should have proven the point, but the battle rages on.

Indications from the F.D.A. point they are considering removing *ALL* amino acids from the public, and making them available *only* with a prescription. This means an office visit plus a cost increase of 500% from pharmaceutical industry. Amino acids are the components of proteins. If the F.D.A succeeds with this they might well take away all nutrients.

I took tryptophan for years when it was available. I never saw any problem with my patients nor did I have any myself. If tryptophan is _so unsafe,_ why is it added to every baby formula on the market. If tryptophan becomes a drug, we have lost the battle to Big Brother, God Help Us!

It is important to let your elected representatives in Washington know how you feel. Write, call and visit them. Congress controls the F.D.A., and we should have the freedom to choose natural instead of legalized addictive prescription drugs.

Sleep / Nighttime Difficulties

Deviations from normal sleep patterns, strange eating habits and allergies frequently appear together in the hyperactive / learning disabled. Sometimes improving the diet will relieve the sleep pathology. Consider halting milk ingestion to allow comfortable sleep without bedwetting. Additionally, the phlegm in the nose may dry up. Sleep is a biochemical phenomenon, but emotional influences can change sleep patterns. Sleep resistance, or the inability to fall asleep in 20 minutes is often due to a deficiency of calcium, magnesium or manganese. A sugary dessert may make the blood sugar fall then an adrenalin release would preclude sleep.

Restless sleep or constant wakefulness, often accompanied by bad dreams or terrors, are usually the result of falling blood sugar and adrenalin release, plus a low serotonin level. The symptoms would be the 120 pulse rate, dilated pupils and generalized perspiration. These are caused by adrenalin, not anxiety. The adrenalin makes a normal dream a scary or terrifying one.

Nutritional Support Program for Hyperactivity / A.D.D.

The following is the program used by the Pain & Stress Therapy Center in San Antonio.

1. Kids Plex, Jr. formula contains the amino acids that activate the neurotransmitters in the brain. Kids Plex mixes with fruit juice and aids the child by providing 100 percent absorption of the needed nutrients.

2. Calms Kids, an amino acid complex for hyperactive and A.D.D. children.

3. AM-PM Plus, a total formula effective in quieting the hyperactive child. AM-PM Plus can be used for daytime hyperactivity, stress or anxiety at night to quiet the child prior to bed.

4. Glutamine, a free form amino acid, found to be deficient in hyperactive and A.D.D. children.

5. Cal, Mag, Zinc, a special synergistic combination of calcium, magnesium and zinc for maximum absorption.

6. Taurine, a free form amino acid, is needed for proper growth and brain function.

7. Glycine, a free form amino acid and is one of the most important neurotransmitters. It can be used without worry of adverse side effects by sprinkling on food as a substitute for sugar. Glycine assists in calming aggressive hyperactive behavior.

8. Reishi mushroom is beneficial to those with allergic reactions, both food and airborne.

9. Gymnema Sylvestre helps in controlling sugar craving in children and adults.

10. TotalVite, a one a day multi-mineral vitamin, provides the body with all of the basic nutrients.

Self Help Products

For a free catalog of products, cassette tapes and books, write:

Pain & Stress Therapy Center
5282 Medical Drive, Suite 160
San Antonio, TX 78229
OR
Call 1-800-669-CALM.

For more information, read or listen to the following:

Books:

The Anxiety Epidemic (Dr. Billie J. Sahley)	$ 9.95
Breaking Your Addiction Habit (Drs. Billie J. Sahley and Katherine M. Birkner)	$ 8.95
Breaking The Sugar Addiction Cookbook (Kathy Birkner, C.R.N.A., Ph.D.)	$ 5.95
Chronic Emotional Fatigue (Dr. Billie J. Sahley)	$ 3.95
Is This Your Child? (Dr. Doris Rapp)	$12.95
Allergies & Your Family (Dr. Doris Rapp)	$12.95
Food Allergies Made Simple (Phylis Austin, et al)	$ 4.95
Toxic Parents (Dr. Susan Forward)	$ 5.95

Tapes:

Hyperactivity-A.D.D. Causes & Control (Dr. Billie J. Sahley)	$10.95
Panic & Anxiety Attacks (Dr. Billie J. Sahley)	$10.95
Environmental Aspects of Allergy (Dr. Doris Rapp)	$10.95
Allergy Diet (Dr. Doris Rapp)	$10.95
Infant Food Allergies (Dr. Doris Rapp)	$10.95
Anxiety (Dr. Billie J. Sahley)	$ 9.95
Building Childrens' Self Esteem (Stephanie Marston)	$ 9.95
Discipline With Love (Stephanie Marston)	$ 9.95

Orthomolecular Consults

If you are unable to find an orthomolecular therapist in your area and would like assistance with a program for yourself or your child, the Pain & Stress Therapy Center provides this service. Phone consultations are available via long distance to help you with a complete program. Information is sent to you in advance to fill out and return prior to the appointment.

If you have any questions or would like to set up an appointment, call the Pain & Stress Center office at (210) 614-7246 weekdays.

Bibliography

Adams, Ruth and Murray, Frank. *Megavitamin Therapy.* New-
York: Larchmont Books, 1980.

American Journal of Disease of Children, December 16-21, 1985.

Austin, Phylis, Thrash, Agatha, and Thrash, Calvin. *Food Allergies Made Simple.* Seale, AL: New Lifestyle Books,
1985.

Bland, Jeffrey. *Medical Applications of Clinical Nutrition.* New
Canaan, Conn: Keats Publishing, Inc., 1983.

Carey, William B. "A Suggested Solution to the Confusion in
Attention Deficit Diagnoses." *Clinical Pediatrics.* Vol.
27, No. 7, July, 1988, pp. 348-349.

Children's Health. (Entire Issue) "Complementary Medicine." Vol.
3, No. 2., Winter, 1988.

Cohen, Sidney. *The Chemical Brain, The Neurochemistry of Addictive Disorders.* Irvine, CA: Care Institute, 1988.

Cooper, Jack R., Bloom, Floyd E., and Roth, Robert H. *The
Biochemical Basis of Neuropharmacology.* New York:
Oxford University Press, 1986.

Cott, Allan. *The Orthomolecular Approach to Learning Disabilities.* Novato, CA: Academic Therapy Publications, 1977.

Cott, Allan with Agel, Jerome, and Boe, Eugene. *Dr. Cott's Help
Your Learning Disabled Child.* New York: Times Books,
Random House, 1985.

Crook, William G. *Allergy and How it Affects You and Your
Child.* Jackson, TN: Professional Books, 1984.

Crook, William G. and Laura Stevens. *Solving the Puzzle of Your
Hard-To-Raise Child.* New York: Vintage Books, 1988.

Essman, W.B., ed. *Nutrients and Brain Function.* New York:
Karger Publishers, 1987.

Feingold, Ben F. *Why Your Child is Hyperactive.* New York:
Random House, 1974.

Grollman, Earl A. *Talking About Death.* Boston: Beacon Press,
1976.

Hamburg, Beatrix A. "Early Adolescence." *Postgraduate Medicine,*
Vol. 78, No. 1, July, 1985, pp. 158-172.

Hoffer, Abram, and Walker, Morton. *Orthomolecular Nutrition New Lifestyle for Super Good Health.* New Canaan, Conn: Keats Publishing, Inc., 1978.

Irwin, M., Belendiuk, K., McCloskey, K., et al. " Tryptophan Metabolism in Children with Attentional Deficit Disorder." *American Journal of Psychiatry.* Vol. 138, No. 8, pp. 1082-1085.

Martin, Paul. "Helping for the Learning Disabled." *Health Express,* June, 1983, pp. 78-79.

New York Times, May 5, 1987, p. 3.

Pheiffer, Carl. *Nutrition and Mental Illness, An Orthomolecular Approach to Balancing Body Chemistry.* Rochester, VT: Healing Arts Press, 1987.

Phelps, Janice Keller and Nourse, Alan E. *The Hidden Addiction and How to Get Free.* Boston: Little, Brown and Company, 1986.

Podell, Richard N. "Food, Mind, and Mood, Hyperactivity Revisited." *Postgraduate Medicine.* Vol. 78, No. 2, August, 1985, pp. 119-125.

Rapp. Doris J. *Allergies and the Hyperactive Child.* New York: Simon and Schuster, Inc. 1979.

Rapp, Doris J. *Is This Your Child?* New York: William Morrow and Company, Inc. 1991.

Renshaw, Domeena. *The Hyperactive Child.* New York: Little and Brown Company, 1974.

The Reporter Weekly. September 2, 1987, p. 10.

Safer, D.J. and Krager, J.M. "A Survey of Medication Treatment for Hyperactive/Inattentive Students." *Journal of theAmerican Medical Association,* October 21, 1988, Vol. 260, No. 15, pp. 2256-2258.

Sahley, Billie. *The Anxiety Epidemic.* San Antonio, TX: Watercrest Press, 1986.

Shaywitz, S.E. and Shaywitz, B.A. "Increased Medication Use in Attention-Deficit Hyperactivity Disorder: Regressive or Appropriate?" *Journal of the American Medical Association,* October 21, 1988, Vol. 260, No. 15, pp. 2270-2272.

Shute, Wilfrid. *Health Preserver, Defining the Versatility of Vitamin E.* Emmanus, PA: Rodale Press, 1977.

Smith, Lendon. *Feed Your Kids Right.* New York: Dell Publishing, 1988.

Smith, Lendon. *Improving Your Child's Behavior Chemistry.* New York: Simon & Schuster, 1977.

Stewart, Mark. *Raising A Hyperactive Child.* New York: Harper Row, 1973.

USA Today. Newslines. October 28, 1988, Section A, p.1.

Williams, Roger. *Biochemical Individuality.* Austin, TX: University of Texas Press, 1979.

Wunderlich, Ray C, Jr. and Kalita, Dwight K. *Nourishing Your Child A Bioecologic Approach*, New Canaan, Conn.: Keats Publishing, Inc., 1984.

Rx For Disease

The greatest disease of mankind is a lack of love for children, leading to their psychological and sometimes, even physical abuse which predisposes those children to a hopeless-helpless attitude, and to disease later in life. We cannot keep blaming physical poisons or genetic defects for every disease. We have to realize that there are poisons in our own homes that predispose us to disease by creating certain attitudes and feelings within us.

Dr. Billie J. Sahley

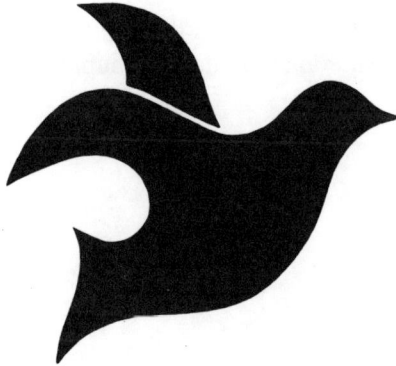

About the Author

Billie J. Sahley, Ph.D. is Executive Director of the Pain & Stress Therapy Center in San Antonio, Texas. She is a Board Certified Medical Psychotherapist and Orthomolecular Therapist. She is a Diplomate in American Academy of Pain Management. Dr. Sahley is a graduate of the University of Texas, Clayton University School of Behavioral Medicine, and U.C.L.A. School of Integral Medicine. Additionally, she has studied advanced nutritional biochemistry through Jeffrey Bland, Ph.D. and HealthComm. She is a member of the Huxley Foundation, Academy of Psychosomatic Medicine, American Academy of Pain Management, Sports Medicine Foundation, American Association of Hypnotherapist, and American Mental Health Counselors Association. Dr. Sahley is also on the Scientific and Medical Advisory Board for Inter-Cal Corporation. She is author of *The Anxiety Epidemic* and *Chronic Emotional Fatigue,* co-author of *Breaking Your Addiction Habit,* and numerous audio cassette tapes.